If My
HOO-HAH
Could Talk

Tips and Tricks for Men
and the Women They Want to Please

Elisabet

TABLE OF CONTENTS

INTRODUCTION

Many of us enter onto the field where sex is played – our bodies and our minds – with absolutely no clue.

Does anyone understand how a body that's not yours actually works?

How could you without doing some homework, or just asking your partner?

Sadly, we often don't ask, and sex becomes a routine we follow and hope for the best. We've become lazy. This isn't just men; women also need to learn the man's body and his needs.

What feels good to body parts you don't have? Do you want to know what does? Done the right way, this research is fun and beneficial.

We think sex or lovemaking is an instinct we're born with. It isn't. Some people are naturally sexy and have a good instinct about what to do. But what about the ones who don't?

After many years of listening to both men and women complain about their sex partners, I can say that the number of experienced and talented lovers is small and getting smaller since we've entered the age of social media. We've forgotten how to romance. Internet dating has become so impersonal. Everything is based on what people have written about themselves, which in turn is based on how they think they look or used to look. How many show up for the first date looking nothing like their dating website picture? How much is the real person, and how much was a sales pitch to get you to contact them?

Most of the pictures displayed are false representations of what the person looks like now. When you finally meet this person, you have an image of what they're going to be. Then you sit before the real person, and guess what, it isn't.

I'm sure there are some good endings to internet dating, and some people do find that special someone. But I assure you it happens only because the couple kept dating and got to know each other.

Some people have instant chemistry, and if this happens for you, great. It's a sadly small percentage, though, because it takes time to develop a relationship.

Understanding someone's needs sexually and emotionally takes time.

Becoming a good and skilled lover takes time,

patience, and the willingness to learn and accept constructive feedback.

Why take someone's request as a criticism if it's something you don't know? Don't be offended if your partner tries to give you guidance on their likes and dislikes!

When you start school or a new job, you hear criticism and get evaluated on a regular basis. You take this in stride and feel it's helping you to do better. You try to improve the bad grade or evaluation to maintain a good grade point average or keep your job, because it's important to you and you want to do well. Why should sex be any different?

Some of us aren't good communicators, so it can be awkward. But you can easily learn about your partner with books, the Internet, good friends, or family you feel comfortable with. Of course, the best source is your partner, because what feels good to one person can be a complete turn-off to another.

It may feel uncomfortable at first, but imagine if he or she also wants to go to this place, and by opening the door you've set the relationship free of this limitation! Don't expect to solve everything at once, but if you can open that door and get him or her to understand some of your needs, you've made progress.

As men and women get older, they become more experienced – but so many of us get into bad habits that become second nature! If a man or woman is never told that something he or she is doing is more annoying than pleasurable, they'll incorporate this "move" into their repertoire. Unbeknownst to them, they'll develop the reputation of a bad lover.

When you stop to think about it, what or who prepares us for the sexual experience? Almost no one!

Some women have an advantage: they ask questions and aren't afraid to say they don't know much about the subject. Women share stories and actual experiences, in full detail.

Men are more cautious about letting anyone know they don't understand the requirements for being a good sexual partner. Men get together and boast on great lovemaking they may have had. But when is the last time you and your buddies exchanged techniques or asked for sexual advice? Women do it more often – though this alone does not make them better lovers.

I had a friend who sadly told me that at the age of 26 she'd never had an orgasm. I asked her if she masturbated; she seemed embarrassed at first by my question, but answered that she never had. I explained that if *she* didn't know how to satisfy herself, how could she expect anyone else to?

When a woman is having sex with a man, he is in many ways a prop like a vibrator or whatever else she might use to climax. Hopefully he's a lot more fun, but you're still using his body to satisfy yourself. Having knowledge of how to do this helps!

Months later my friend confessed that I changed her sex life: she was having great orgasms and enjoying sex for the first time.

If a man is really good, we women might describe to close friends or relatives what he did and how it made us feel. The not-so-good ones get even more attention and descriptions of all their lousy moves.

I'm sure the female population could use help in the sex arena, and of course a lot of gals keep their thoughts to themselves, but I want to focus on the male situation. This is not meant to attack men and put the entire burden on them. But as a woman, I know the things that are lacking from a woman's perspective. I hope to give some tips on things that men may just not be thinking to do or say.

At some young age, boys start to get erections, and sooner or later start to masturbate. It's rare that anyone explains all that can be done with their magic wand or that there's more to sex than just an erection. The male organ is quite simple sexually because it's out in the open. I know it has sensitive areas and not-as-sensitive areas, and, like any part of the human body, responds better to certain things. I know men would love for women to have an understanding of their manhood, and I hope to shed some light on that subject.

On the other hand, women have a lot going on down there! No instructions come with us, so our partners have to fly by the seat of their pants and hope that something they're doing is hitting the mark.

We all rely on instructions when we can't figure out the working parts of something. This book is a simple guide; it isn't the answer to all the sexual problems between men and women, but it's a start!

This is not a medical guide or in any way a substitute for professional help. Should you have medical needs, please seek a doctor or therapist. This book is just for clean fun and some pointers to enjoying sex. It requires a healthy mind and body. I am not a doctor and do not give medical advice. The advice is for healthy males with no sexual medical problems. If you suffer from a sexual dysfunction I highly recommend you see a physician. There have been some wonderful new discoveries in this area and your problem may not be as bad as you think.

All the blame certainly does not belong to the men. I realize that women can also be bad lovers. I'm writing this from the female experience; hopefully, some knowledgeable male will step up to the plate and enlighten women on what men like. If it could help women to understand the working parts of something we don't have (a penis), I'd be all for it.

I write this book to explain from one woman's experience what some women need, and hopefully to pass on some helpful hints on how to become a better lover. This is only an opinion and has no medical bearing. This information is also based on many years of one-on-one conversations with other women who have shared their sexual disappointments and sexual thrills.

We always seem to be complaining about the same thing. Lack of knowledge or experience is most likely the cause. Perhaps calling someone a "bad lover" is unfair. Maybe it's just lack of knowledge in a field most people are too intimidated or embarrassed to inquire about!

All the education you've gotten over the years since high school is about how our organs work, but no one ever goes into detail about how to please us. Sometimes parents give you the facts of life, some good advice, and hopefully some moral education. But many parents don't feel comfortable on the subject, and formal education isn't required to offer instruction (in fact, is generally required *not* to!).

So you got the hot car but don't know that gas makes it run!

In this book, all the subjects will be simple but to the point.

I shared the guide I'm about to give you with a male friend who admitted he needed help in bed. He was having a lady over for the evening, and knew something was missing in their sex life. I told him to get out pencil and paper and take notes. I promised that his lady would be begging him to take her. He confessed this had never happened to him before, and said he'd believe it when he experienced it! This man was thirty years old, and admitted he'd never gotten any woman so hot that she'd screamed with passion for more. He wasn't even sure if they were having orgasms. He'd recently been dumped, and I'm sure lack of sexual performance was a key player.

A few days later he called so ecstatically! He wanted to know more. Once he let his guard down and could accept some tips, his sex life improved.

Why did he feel he could share his needs and lack of knowledge with me, but not with his lady? He could have gone to any bookstore and purchased a book on the subject, but he needed a quick fix. We had never had sex, so he was comfortable letting his guard down, knowing I did not know how bad it was, or what other issues he may have had. Since I couldn't judge him, he had nothing to lose. He relaxed and got great advice, and I'm sure his lady must have wondered what happened!

Lots of self-help books on sex go into a great deal of research, or discuss too many topics. If you bought a new lawn mower and had to put it together, you'd want the instructions to be precise and to the point, without any extra parts you have no idea what they're for.

I hope to do that for you in this book. You can pick a chapter that you feel you need help with and read it quickly.

So much of sex is mental and enlightened by all of our senses: touch, sight, smell, and hearing. I will go into subjects that affect these things. They all play a role in our game of sex, because the brain is where a good healthy sex life begins.

So pour yourself a cup of coffee, get in your most comfortable chair, and let's have some good ol' girl talk!

1

PERFORMANCE

That word alone – "performance" – puts a lot of pressure on a man. Let's face it: the man is the one required to perform. Mother Nature tagged you with this responsibility. I will admit it isn't always fair, but that's the set-up. As a man, you're supposed to be the pursuer. Take charge and sweep us off our feet. As corny as it all may seem, it's how it's always been perceived.

Yet over the years, with all the women's liberation movements, the messages sent to men have gotten confusing. Women have become more aggressive and bold. Some men like this, and some men may be intimidated by the aggression. But the bottom line is that most women love romance and appreciate a good skilled lover, no matter who initiated the relationship.

I agree that too much burden is put on the man and that there are a lot of women out there who just plain stink in bed. But right now we're talking about male performance – and you never know, if you're really good maybe you'll warm up a few of those ice maidens! You might even find that after reading this, you'll become a bit more forward about your needs. Because if anyone doesn't want to hear your desires, I say move on. If they're a selfish lover, you most likely will never change that closed mind. Legs may be open, but if the mind is closed, how great do you think things can become?

Remember when you were a teenager and all you were doing was making out, bumping and grinding? All that felt good, and you and your partner were so hot that if you'd been consenting sexual adults, you'd have been all over it (and maybe you were!).

What makes those days so different from now?

First, that was all that you could do, and you were trying hard and hoping this would be the one to take you out of virginity or add to your collection of partners. I remember a lot of good kissing and the feel of the male body rubbing against me. All the sensations felt foreign, but also wonderful.

On many occasions I was having orgasms from passionate make-out sessions, yet when I had actual intercourse, I could not orgasm for months. I had been masturbating for years, so I knew how to please myself.

Why wasn't it happening during the real deal?

Because my lover wasn't in the know of what I needed. We went from slow make out sessions to slam bam, thank you ma'am.

I know a lot of you are saying "I don't do this!", but a large population of you does – even if you could never bring yourself to admit you fall into this category. It sounds selfish and says you don't know what you're doing.

Before you were allowed into the unknown, you took your time, sometimes for hours. As we get older, we don't sit around and make out because we can indulge in the real deal, but why forget what felt so good and worked?

Finally getting to first base is great and also maybe a little scary, simply because you've never been there. Will you come too fast or be really bad? If it's your first time seeing or feeling a vagina, it can be intimidating since you don't understand the working parts.

Women require more time sexually. The male organ is so exposed, and it's very easy to manipulate. The female organ is engulfed in many parts and layers. Knowing where they are and what makes them feel good is so important to being a good lover.

Some men are passionate and good kissers and seem to be performing well until the actual event takes place. Just because you know what's coming, don't stop putting in the effort. Don't be intimidated by the vagina. Touch it, explore the unknown, and make sure you know what you're doing. Put some effort into your new subject. Go online and look up the vagina. I knew a young man that thought the clitoris was inside the vagina. How many satisfied lovers do you think he had? He was shocked when I described its location. So get informed.

Begin your lovemaking with slow passionate kisses; keep them soft and tender. Kiss her face, eyes, and neck. Take your time; it doesn't have to be for hours, but not for five minutes either. You'll sense when the time is right to move on by how turned on you both are. Read your lady's body language; it will tell you what to do and when. (Body language is discussed in chapter 4.)

Be careful not to go any lower than the neck at this point. Slowly seduce her with your kisses. So much of the passion is in kissing. If a person is a stiff hard kisser, most likely the rest of his performance will be too. Women love it when a man is a good kisser – this is something we'll share with friends.

You'll be able to feel her getting aroused. Continue with kissing and incorporate one more move: slowly start to caress her arms, running your fingers long and slowly up and down the full length of her arms. The inside of a woman's arm is very sensitive and can be as arousing as touching her breasts. Slowly run your fingers on the inside of her arm, especially around the inner elbow. This is an area most men never go near, and what a surprise your lady will have when she discovers how incredible this new untouched area feels.

Caressing should be like a feather moving along her body. Close your eyes for a moment and imagine what feels good to you. Feathery soft touching is much more appealing to the body. You're trying to seduce her without ever entering or even touching her vagina at this point. The amount of tenderness she's feeling is not only a turn-on, but also relaxing and hypnotic. Slowly she will surrender to your touches and wonderful knowledge of her body.

Feel the silky skin on her back. There are many nerve endings on the back, so kissing or lightly caressing this area is a great, soothing feeling. If your lady seems a bit uptight, gently rubbing her back could be the key to breaking down her barrier.

Take your caressing a step further and come close to her breasts. Just lightly tease them – it's not a massage. Women's breasts are not balls of dough; they don't require kneading. You can become a bit more aggressive later; right now we are trying to get her hot, hot, hot. Keep in mind teasing is better achieved with slow sensuous moves than harsh, aggressive, clumsy ones.

Move your kissing down close to her breast, lightly licking one of her nipples. Kisses for different parts of the body change, so swirl your tongue around one of her nipples. Mix around your kissing with light sucking and licks to the same nipple. With your other hand, gently tease the other breast. Both nipples will be erect now and begging for more, but hold back. Kiss her gently on the mouth and move your hand down her inner thigh, again with long feathery fingers. Never forget the power of the kiss; it's what got this ball rolling, so go back and kiss her with more passion.

Move your hand down from her breasts along her stomach and start to explore the insides of her thighs. Change from one thigh to another, each time coming closer to her vagina, but not touching it. When you can sense that she is pretty aroused, gently brush over her vagina. Lightly brush over her pubic hair. Lightly touching and gently pulling her pubic hair sends little sensations through her vagina.

Keep your touch to the vaginal area soft and delicate. Touch her clitoris gently at first and slowly apply pressure. Remember, the clitoris is the female penis. It gets aroused and hard just like a penis, and in most women it's what brings on an orgasm. When it's soft, banging on it or touching it roughly isn't going to get you a good response. Imagine if your penis was flaccid and your lady began to bang on it! This would not only be a turn-off, but the purpose of getting you aroused would be defeated. Most likely you would become annoyed at her lack of experience or knowledge about your penis. Not much would happen until it was fully erect, and even then, you don't want your penis treated roughly. Your penis doesn't work until it's ready.

The female anatomy isn't any different. Most men think that just because the actual act takes place inside, the outside doesn't have to be primed. Well, think again! Feel her clitoris gently; it should start to feel harder and larger. Blood is flowing to it just like an erect penis. This is a warm and sensuous feeling, and it will make her want what's coming that much more. Make her desire what you aren't giving her.

Now move your fingers down to the opening of her vagina and slowly start to feel her inside. If you've been doing everything right up to now, she should be wet. Move slowly inside of her with your finger, keeping your thumb rubbing on the nub of her clitoris.

By this time she should be screaming for you to enter her. Slowly bring your body onto hers. Lightly brush your erect penis against her vagina. The feeling of your arousal will enhance hers. She's been waiting to feel what you just did, so the response should be great. Don't be too quick to enter her. Start to kiss her again with more passion. As you're both very aroused now, your movements can be a bit more aggressive, but not hard. She will be dying for you to enter her, and if you have a vocal lady she will be begging you to give her all that you have.

While kissing her, grind your erection against her, applying just the right amount of pressure – very similar to dry humping when you were too young to have sex. Slowly start to enter her vagina. She will be craving for more, but remember not giving her what she wants will enhance her desire. The penis entering the vagina can be very sensuous, so play this up. The skin on the penis feels like no other skin, especially when rubbed onto a vagina. Since no skin is ever rubbed down there (except her fingers!), the penis is a foreign feel that, used properly, is amazing. Slowly moving with just the head of your penis inside her is a great tease. Give her only enough to let her feel what's coming.

Now that you've fully entered her, move in a nice rhythm that flows. She should greet each of your movements with her body. Pay attention to her movements; they will guide you on how much she needs or wants. Learn to listen with your body. If she's being aggressive, then follow her lead, but if she's moving slowly, she wants to be taken nice and slow.

You're in the dance of passion; try to stay together in your movements. Try not to be doing the two-step when she's doing the rumba. If you feel that going harder is what your lady desires then do so, but remember that banging into us like a jackhammer can be a turn-off. The vaginal area is delicate and soft, so hard banging for some women is unpleasant. If your lady screams "harder," then go for it, but remember to read her body language; it will tell you how to proceed.

Lovemaking is like a snowball rolling down a hill: it builds up speed and gets bigger as it moves. Allow things to grow according to the mood. Once you feel your lady start to orgasm, don't push too hard into her clitoris; in some women this stops their flow. Don't talk during this time either, unless it's been part of your game. Moans or screams should be the only sounds at this climatic time.

It's important to try to feel what your lady needs and when she needs it. I know this may sound complicated, but if you just pay attention and let things flow you'll get a lesson every time you make love – and after a while you'll begin to understand and feel her needs. Things should flow pretty smoothly from here.

I'll discuss oral sex and other methods of teasing in other chapters. This is just a basic plan for intercourse. There are so many things to try and adventures to take when making love, but they're generally a personal preference. If something is working for you and your partner, don't let someone else intimidate you into thinking that what they do is the bomb of all sexual experiences. We're all different and our views on sex differ, so if it feels good, go with it. Sex doesn't have to be complicated or confused with more being better. If different positions are something you enjoy, then incorporate them into your lovemaking, but make sure your partner likes them as well.

The art of lovemaking is about pleasing each other and trying to find out what your partner likes.

2

SIZE

This is a touchy subject, but one that has to be addressed.

When you hear that size doesn't matter, for a penis-oriented woman, it is going to matter.

Some women like to feel fullness and need penetration to climax, while other women are into cunnilingus and it's their preference or even the only way that they can climax. Look at all the lesbians out there; they certainly have mastered the use of sexual objects and the power of the tongue.

If you have a small penis, learn to work around it, and try to find a woman who loves cunnilingus.

That said, most of your problems will be in your mind and will most likely hamper your performance. Most women would rather have a man with a small penis than one who comes too soon. Don't allow your ego to get in the way. Be adventuresome. You know your penis is small, so introduce toys. Make up for size with passion. Ask your lady what she wants. Women love when men care enough to see to their needs.

Now for those who have a really large penis, first of all be grateful, and secondly, learn how to use it. You don't generally hear much complaining about these guys except when they don't know how to use what nature has given them. Nothing is more disappointing to a woman than to get a nicely endowed lover and it all goes to waste. Make sure to follow the plan in chapter 1 and let the rest fall into place.

Some women do have a small vagina, so a large penis can be a problem. If this is the case, be considerate of your lady and take it easy. She will let you know when enough is enough.

The one women dislike the most is the bragger. If you don't have the performance to back up the goods, keep your mouth shut. Women don't go around bragging about their vaginas – they don't have to! So imagine how a woman feels when you step up to the plate and strike out. Stay low-key and let your performance speak for itself. It never fails: the guy who brags the most is generally the worst in bed.

I have a friend whom a man had pursued for years to go to bed with him. He bragged about how he would rock her world. During one evening of drinking, and tired of listening to him boast, she gave in, hoping he would be all that he'd professed. Not only did he come in three seconds – his foreplay had an even shorter shelf life. She was so angry she turned to him and said, "Is that it, after all of these years of bragging, that's your best shot?" Needless to say he stormed out of the room and never spoke to her again. She may have been cruel, but he deserved it. I bet he'll think twice about ever boasting again about his great manly talents! Hopefully he'll read this book and pick up a few tips.

Interesting, though: she never mentioned the size of his penis, just what a bad lover he was. So while size plays an important role for many women, most women like tenderness, passion, and a skilled, considerate lover. In the end, it's all about what you're able to deliver.

3

TALK THE TALK

Sex talk can be very arousing and great foreplay when done correctly. Sex talk can be done in person, over the phone, in a note, or through body language. It does not have to be vulgar. You can be nasty and still keep it clean. It's done all the time in romance novels where the author describes the lovemaking between the two characters and sparks are flying everywhere. These books tend to be written with beauty and a lot of suggestive writing – you certainly get the message about what's going on!

The choice of words is entirely up to you and what you think your partner will respond to. Use common sense. If the lady you're trying to entice is a bit of a prude, coming on with heavy four-letter words may scare her off. This doesn't mean you can't use sex talk with her – just watch how you approach it. And when she gets really hot, I'm sure no four-letter word will matter!

When you're making love, remember to lower your voice. I can't stress this point enough. When talking to someone sexually, you don't want to sound like you're delivering a sales pitch or ordering a rum and coke in a crowded bar. Lovemaking is a quiet sort of hypnotic moment. A loud burst of your voice could disturb the ambiance. Your voice should soften and become a little husky. Put passion into your words. No baby-talk, either. This is such a turn-off, and even if it's cute in the beginning, it will eventually sound stupid.

Begin the seduction with sex talk before you ever get to the plan in chapter 1. Let your words be breathy. This is good when you are close to her ear. The heat of your breath plus the words are arousing.

Don't be repetitive; instead, try to be creative. You can base your sex talk around compliments, but keep it honest. Don't make outlandish remarks that you know she won't believe. Try to remember the things that drive her crazy and replay them for her. Turn it into a fantasy, letting the two of you be the characters. Remember a place you've been together and fantasize with her that you had the urge to take her right then and there. If this is a first-time event, talk to her about how you've been fantasizing about her and tell her things that you thought of doing should you ever get the chance. Include her in the escapade by asking her questions. Does she want this or that done to her? Before you know it, she'll be asking you questions and playing right along in this fun sexual game.

The bedroom is the adult playroom, but it doesn't have to start there. While out to dinner, make sexual suggestions and start the ball rolling. There are so many things that can work for you. Don't be shy! Try one and see where it goes.

On the other hand, too much talking can be a turn-off. An important rule to remember is when to stop talking and get some action going. A good time to clam up is when she is into her climax. Your voice could change or ruin the fantasy she has going on in her mind.

If you've tried sex talk and feel uncomfortable with it, try phone sex; it might be easier if you aren't face to face with the person. Practice when you're alone. A good time would be during masturbation. Think of how your imagination works when you're alone trying to get aroused.

If you travel a lot, phone sex is great. Just remember to keep your voice low and husky, which sounds even better over the phone. After all, when a woman gets an obscene phone call, the caller is generally a heavy breather. While these types of phone calls are not appreciated, the pervert knows that breathing is part of the act.

Tell her all the great things you plan on doing to her when you get home. Go over chapter 1 in your mind and relive it for her on the phone. Describe your last lovemaking session and how much you've missed her.

Again, ask her questions about herself. You may unleash a tiger you didn't know existed.

Since all you have is your imagination, vivid descriptions can be very tantalizing. The only picture you have is the one painted for you. Your guard is down, and a fantasy begins that could get very intense. Try it some time. It could improve your sex life, because you could relive the phone sex all over again when you get together.

Writing is something you have to achieve on your own, but you're either good with words or you're not, so if you're not much of a writer, stay away from this one. Sending an already-printed card can be sweet and thoughtful. Many card shops are now carrying adult material, so let someone else be creative and sign your name to it. The message will be the same.

Whether you write it or you buy a pre-written card, placing the note in interesting places is always fun and a great surprise. Be romantic. Include a flower with it. Going the extra mile doesn't have to be complicated or expensive. Spray her favorite cologne that you wear on the card. I know some women who, when their man is away, they'll smell his favorite shirt just to have a quick reminder of him.

Little things like this are always good to do after a great session of lovemaking, or if you're trying to get one started. I promise your thoughtfulness will stay with her most of the day. Most women are hopeless romantics. We eat it up when a man is romantic. So little effort goes into being romantic, but for some reason we all become a little lazy and stop putting in the effort. There are some wonderful books on romantic things to do. If you can't be creative on your own, invest in one of these helpful guides.

4

BODY LANGUAGE

Body language is something you have to look for and understand. We'd need a psychiatrist educated on body movement to interpret and diagnose most of it, so let's just talk about the moves involving sexual suggestion.

Body language, like any other language, can also be a turn-off. Try not to come on too strong with your body. I have a friend who moves in very close when she meets a man. When I observe this, I find most of the men lean back to regain their space.

Moving in like this may be appropriate after you've known someone, but for the first introduction it can be too aggressive. If you don't read body language correctly and give off the proper message, you'll receive a bad response, just like my friend! Pay attention to the way the body moves.

Both men and women will make suggestions with their eyes and mouth. Something as subtle as parting the lips and licking them can be suggestive. Have you ever seen a woman walk into a room and her walk transfixed every man who could see her? I can assure you this lady not only knows her walk is powerful; it's one of her signature lures.

During sex the body says so much if you feel for it. If a woman responds to your touches and moves with you, chances are she wants what you want. Remember the plan: in chapter 1 described about when to move forward from one section of the body to the other. Body language will give you most of these answers.

The body's movements during sex are quite beautiful, like a dance. Pay attention to her breathing and sighing; these are good indicators that she's turned on. Not all people are vocal, so rely on movement and breath. Hopefully all your movements will be met with a complimentary rhythm.

You'll also be able to determine her level of arousal by other things like her kissing, how she's touching you, and her willingness to be involved. When she kisses you, is she kissing you with her whole body, or is she stiff? If after doing all your moves she lies there like a dead fish, either she *is* a dead fish, or – more likely – not ready. Some ladies take longer than others to get going. Be patient.

At the same time, understand, gentlemen, you

aren't always going to be a success sexually even with this guide. It takes two and sometimes your partner just stinks in bed. A prudish lover is someone who has led a conservative life.

I had a friend whose boyfriend was raised in a very religious home, so he thought sex was dirty. These types of people need counseling, and unless you are a professional, move on. Sadly, my friend started to feel something was wrong with her. Don't allow someone else's baggage to fall on you. Look for the signs and if the person seems off, move on.

5

HYGIENE

Now, I know you're thinking you don't need someone telling you how to stay clean. Well – wrong! You guys have to stop thinking that only the vagina comes with odors.

What you may not be aware of is that the testicles get musty-smelling, especially if you sweat a lot. Your organs are trapped in pants and underwear all day. Some odor is going to happen.

Some men, no matter how much they bathe, have a musty odor. Some women have this same problem. The best suggestion I can give you is to keep "baby wipes" handy. Make sure to buy organic ones; some have a preservative called methochloroisothiazolinone or MCI/MI. These types of wipes can cause a rash or irritate your skin. I use the organic ones and never have a problem. They are great for a quick clean-up or if you just want to feel fresh.

The worst of all offenders is probably breath. This is becoming the number one turn-off. I have more friends complain about bad breath than anything else. It kills the mood for snuggling or kissing.

If you have bad breath, chances are no one has the courage to tell you. You should be able to tell by the amount of social life you have. If you're married or in a relationship and kissing is non-existent, maybe you should ask your partner if you have breath issues.

If you're not going to the dentist at least twice a year then start going. Consult with your dentist or your dental hygienist; they'll be honest with you.

Sometimes bad breath comes from your stomach or sinuses. If you have a history of sinus infections, this can cause a bad odor. Or you may have a stomach acid problem. There are new drugs on the market for acid and digestive problems. Consult your physician and your problem could be easily corrected.

Dry mouth can also be a cause of bad breath. There are some good mouthwashes on the market to correct dry mouth, so look into it.

If you have yellowing teeth, get them bleached. A pretty white smile is more desirable. If you aren't flossing, start. The new electric toothbrushes do a much better job than you can with a regular toothbrush; invest in one. Try to keep mints or gum handy, especially if you're a smoker – no one wants to kiss an ashtray!

Hopefully all you gentlemen bathe on a daily basis. If you don't, I can only imagine the last successful date that you had. Wash your hair daily; the scalp can also smell. If you have a dandruff problem, get the correct shampoo. Sometimes a good conditioner will help with a dry scalp. If you're in a relationship, there is no excuse to become lazy and let hygiene go.

Lovemaking is so much about the body, so keep it fresh and inviting. You want someone to desire you. This is tough to do if you smell like an old sock.

Speaking of old socks, some of you have foot odor problems. No matter how much you bathe, your feet stink. Most likely your feet sweat. There are so many new products on the market today for this. Look into some and try out a few, and hopefully this will resolve your problem. During sex feet can be arousing. Massaging or licking and kissing the feet is erotic. Don't eliminate yourself from this treat with stinky feet!

Toenails and fingernails can also be a turn-off. I have a friend who's turned off as soon as she sees her husband's feet. This may seem shallow, but remember: so much of sex is in the mind. Something that seems personally revolting can become a mental picture and have an adverse effect on your desire to make love. Remember phone sex, and how a description can be a powerful tool in sex.

So pay attention to your feet and hands. Have a manicure and pedicure once in a while. Dirty toenails and fingernails are not only a turn-off; it implies you haven't bathed. Besides, when you're in bed with someone, rough, dry feet and hands don't feel good.

I know some of you are in a profession that requires the use of your hands, and roughness comes with the territory. Try applying some good hand cream before indulging and it may help the situation. There are hand scrubs that exfoliate dry dead skin off; try them, and you may be surprised. If you prefer to make your own, put salt or sugar in with your liquid soap and create your own scrub.

If you're a very hairy man, consider trimming things up a bit. Keep the pubic area clean and trim. This is important if you enjoy oral sex. If your body is covered in hair and you're self-consciences about it, look into having waxing done. The new hair laser removal programs can be expensive, but they're more permanent. Keep your eyebrows, nose, and ear hair trimmed. Remember you want to be appealing to someone. If you have hair sticking out everywhere, this will be what your lady will focus on. All of these services can be done at most salons and take only a few moments.

And women love a good smelling man, but please don't overdo the cologne!

I know all of you know at least one person who complains about their lack of a social life, and you wish you could be honest with them. It could be their personal hygiene that's keeping them from a healthy social life. Well, that person could be you. Be objective about yourself and take a good hard look at you. Take pride in how you look and smell, and you'll enjoy the benefits.

6

SETTING THE MOOD

Setting a mood can be fun and romantic.

Have you ever gone to a restaurant or bar and the atmosphere was romantic? The owner did that on purpose. He or she wants you to come relax and get into the mood. If you feel romantic, you'll indulge yourself more.

When my husband proposed to me, he took me to a romantic restaurant. He requested a table by the fire. There were roses on the table with a beautiful card. He set a mood. He wouldn't have thought to propose – or to set a mood! – in some greasy diner.

Moods are an expression of how you want things to go. Be spontaneous – and make plans.

My husband had been gone two long weeks, so when I picked him up at the airport I was wearing next to nothing under a full-length fur coat. He couldn't keep his hands off of me the whole ride home. The mood for my evening had been set at the airport.

Mood settings don't have to be complicated or out of your home. Use what you have around you. Soft, sexy music is always enticing. So is soft lighting. Turn off all electricity and light candles everywhere. Candlelight sets off a warm glow that's easy on the eyes and doesn't have to be altered should things get rolling. Fresh flowers are pretty and send the message that you put in some effort. A good bottle of wine is always a nice touch.

The best prop is you. Wear something sexy. If you happen to look great in a T-shirt and jeans then go for it. And sometimes less is better. Try answering the door in a pair of silk boxers. They're great because when things get steamy silk has a hard time holding down your excitement.

Sexy attire isn't only for women so be creative. Absolutely smell good, but as I said at the end of the last chapter, please don't overdo the cologne.

If your house needs help, do some cleaning. If you're too busy to clean, hire a cleaning lady. You'll be surprised how affordable they are and the time that it will save you!

Think ahead and have fresh towels in the bathrooms. Make sure the bed sheets are clean. If you have pets, try to get the pet hair out of the way and clean up any pet odors. This can be a turn-off, and many people are allergic. The last thing you want is your lady sneezing all night or picking pet hairs off her clothes.

You may love your pet, but give your lady the opportunity to get used to you first. I have a friend whose husband insisted that the dog sleep with them every night. The dog weighed ninety pounds and smelled. How often do you think she gets in a sexy mood? If getting ladies to come back to your place after the first visit is a problem, your place might need some clean-up, or you might have some pet issues.

If you have old photos of an ex sitting around, get rid of them. Why put a damper on the evening with your past staring at her?

If this is a special evening, don't take phone calls, or at least cut them short. It's rude, and you're giving off the message that she can wait. If your profession requires you to be on call sometimes, do your mood evening at time when you're *not* on call. Cell phones are the rudest technology! When did any of us become so important that we have to have a cell phone at all times? If you're not a surgeon with someone's life depending on you, leave your phone off or at home.

Be creative with your mood. Do something differently, like a theme night. The atmosphere should be indicative of the theme. Pick an old movie that you both like and be the characters. Special holidays are always fun to act on. These leave you both with great memories.

If you live together or are married, all the above still applies. Come home a little early and surprise her with a special night. It may put back some of the spark missing from your relationship. One of the problems with relationships today is we get lazy and start taking our passion for granted. When the relationship was new, you thought all those sparks flying came naturally. Well, the reality is that both of you were working harder in the beginning, trying to impress each other. The newness also made things more exciting.

People go out looking for something else because of all the fun and spontaneity that comes with a new relationship. After spending time with this new person, you'll be back in the same boat. Your old relationship most likely started out with the same bang and both of you got lazy. So instead of going out looking for someone new, try doing some of the old things that you used to do – or set a whole new mood! – and see what happens.

A girlfriend of mine recently complained that her husband's birthday was coming up and she had no idea what to buy him. I said, "Why buy him anything? Do a theme night!" Of course she wanted all the details. I gave her some ideas and she got the ball rolling. He came home to a total surprise and could not keep his hands off her. This gift can't be returned, it certainly fits, and I guarantee a second one just like the first would be greatly appreciated!

7

KISSING

Kissing can be so damn sexy and can make your evening of passion. This is where we all started, and yet we cut it short in our foreplay.

Kissing doesn't have to be associated with sex every time. You could meet someone and just be comfortable kissing. After some time if things get hotter, you may want sex, but the kissing up to this point was fun.

I have a male friend who dated a woman who was a bore sexually. He continued to see her because she was fun and happen to be a good kisser. So on most dates they snuggled and made out. Eventually he did move on in search of the whole package, but it was fun for a while.

Kissing is a skill I think most people could do better if taught. I've instructed some men who became very good kissers. The problem is, most people don't know how to come out and tell you that you can't kiss. You end up going through life being tagged the "bad kisser." It's like having to tell someone they have bad breath; we don't want to do it, so we think we'll let the next person tell them, and of course no one ever does.

Something so simple should be quite easy. It comes naturally for some and some never get it. Like lovemaking, kissing is something we all learn along the way. Your parents and teachers never held a class on making out!

There are different types of kisses and all can be nice. A gentle soft kiss on the lips is the general beginning. Keep your lips moist and soft. If you have dry chapped lips, use something on them: no one wants to kiss dry cracked lips. Try applying a lip balm before going to bed and you'll wake up to softer lips. Applying some lip balm before kissing is always good.

To explain the art of kissing, we should discuss what makes really bad kisses. Here are a few examples.

THE MILK BOTTLE. This is when the guy opens his mouth and no tongue is used. It's like kissing a milk bottle. Why bother to open your mouth at all? If this is how you kiss, stick with soft lip kissing until you master French kissing.

If you want to French kiss, try applying some

tongue. You're not trying to swallow her head, so don't open your mouth so wide. Slowly and softly insert your tongue into her mouth and play with her tongue. Keep the tongue soft. A stiff tongue is not for kissing. Imagine the way you would lick something sticky off of your lips: with a soft tongue to get up all of the nice sweetness. Treat kissing with the same feeling. Savor each sensation like you were licking an ice cream cone; and you don't want it to end and give up the delicious treat.

THE DART: This is where the tongue is used, but incorrectly. It shoots in and out of your mouth like a dart or as if you're kissing a snake. If you do this, stop! It's a major indication of how the rest of your performance will be: in and out quickly. Slow down and make kissing passionate. Not doing this is the worst mistake in lovemaking!

THE SLOBBER: This one speaks for itself. No one wants to kiss a bunch of saliva. Try swallowing before you start to kiss. If your kissing partners require a clean-up after kissing you, then you're slobbering.

HARD LIPS: I asked several friends, both male and female, and this was the biggest complaint. Take your hand and move it up to your lips. Kiss it softly and gently. Pretend you're kissing a baby's head. This is what your partner wants to feel.

Now press your lips firmly together and kiss your hand again. This should settle that debate. When French kissing, keep the lips and tongue soft, but careful not to open your mouth too wide. Practice relaxing your mouth. If you have nice full lips, use them to your advantage – big soft lips are so kissable. The act of kissing should come naturally. Relax and go with it.

THE BITER: Some women like this move, but most are turned off by it, especially if you are hard biter. Little nibbles are different from a bite. Always try to find out what your partner likes. Try your technique, and if she continues kissing you, maybe she's into biting. If your lady backs off, then biting is out. Lips are soft and tender, so keep your nibbles gentle; some ladies may find this a turn-on.

THE LICKER: I don't know anyone that enjoys this one. We don't want to feel like we are out with our pets. I have a male friend whose lady would lick around his teeth till he thought he was at the dentist. Small subtle licking can be a turn-on, but face washing is not.

Licking other parts of the body is a great turn-on, but remember that the mouth does not respond like the vagina. Save your licking for the right places and you could be a big success.

How can you become a good kisser who will make your partner want more? If you didn't see yourself in any of these descriptions, chances are you're doing okay. If you have a great success at make-out sessions, you also are doing just fine. But if you happen to see any indication that you may fall into the above categories, then you need help.

Kissing just isn't about the lips and tongue. A really good passionate kiss involves the body. (There goes that body language thing again!) If someone is kissing stiffly with their body and lips, what message are you getting? When you kiss someone, fall into it with everything you have. Feel the passion start at your lips, and let the sensation move down through your body. This can be done even if you're seated. Don't overdo the head movements; stay in rhythm with your partner.

Start off with moist soft lips. Kiss her gently, slowly introducing your tongue. Open your mouth enough to move your tongue comfortably. A wide-open mouth is the beginning of the Milk Bottle kisser. You want to kiss her, not swallow her head. Swirl your tongue around in a nice rhythm. Not too much tongue and not too little, like you're afraid to come in. Keep things moving nicely with a gentle sway to your head and body, but don't over-exaggerate your moves.

If you want to hold her head and run your fingers through her hair, this is a sexy move. Stop occasionally and kiss her face, eyes, and light kisses on the lips before you indulge again. Kiss her lips often, keeping in mind French kissing isn't continual. You kiss with your tongue and then lips again, mixing it up.

Make kissing last as long as you need it. Remember, it's the beginning of a great treat, like a bottle of wine that should be enjoyed slowly. Kissing is such a simple form of foreplay. Enjoy it and savor the many benefits from the simple kiss.

8

HOME BASE

This is where you ultimately want to end up, and hopefully with a home run.

The vagina isn't complicated when you understand all its working parts. Learn what she's all about, and you'll have most of your sexual problems solved.

I agree the female anatomy can be complicated, but it's what nature gave women, so get educated. Think for a moment how it feels to have a woman who really knows how to push all your buttons. You can relax and totally enjoy the moment without feeling like you have to instruct. Just like you, women love it when a man knows his way around home base.

Although there are many parts to the female anatomy, we want to focus on the ones that give her pleasure. If you need a chart or pictures go to the

Internet and look into the female anatomy for a full description.

I imagine that finding the clitoris and G-spot are probably what gives you the most doubt.

First of all, they're not the same. One is on the outside and one is inside. The clitoris is on the outside just below the hood. If you take your finger and go straight down past the pubic bone, you'll feel the clitoris. Press in gently and you'll feel a small nub. Rubbing this with your finger or licking it with your tongue will drive your lady crazy. Be careful not to apply too much pressure: that could either be irritating or even stop her orgasm.

The Grafenberg Spot, also known as the "G" spot, is an area you should locate right away. The orgasm that comes from the G-spot is generally earth-shaking. If you put your finger into her vagina and probe, gently pushing your finger forward toward the navel, you'll hit the G-spot. When you do, your lady will most likely let you know.

This area is sometimes best found if she is on her hands and knees. Rear positions are good because the slight tilt of your penis should hit the G-spot with each thrust. Massaging the G-spot during cunnilingus can also create a great orgasm; just know when to back off pressure so that you don't interfere with her orgasm.

Be patient looking for all these places. She may not even know where her G-spot is. If you feel comfortable with her, ask her to help you out with specific locations. Not everyone likes the same thing, so inquire as to her preference. This may in turn get her to ask you what you like. Wouldn't it be great to have a good sexual communication with your partner?

Don't ignore the labia – the folds or lips of the vagina. Make sure to treat these as gently as if you were kissing her mouth. Light teasing with the tongue in this area is very appealing. Once the clitoris is hard and aroused, your pressure can increase. Learn to feel and sense your lady and she'll be appreciative. Throughout this book the one lesson that goes with everything you do is: slow, gentle, and passionate.

Enjoy your bodies with a good healthy attitude and be open minded and giving to your lover. A selfish lover is one who gets replaced. Explore all your sexuality has to offer, and you'll be rewarded many times over.

9

THE BLOWJOB

Now, ladies, if you're not doing this for your man and it's something he loves, you need to recognize that. I've always said, "Giving a blow job is like eating escargot," because you can't put a lot of thought into it. If you focused only on the fact that you're eating a snail, you wouldn't eat it. Escargot made properly is delicious, so why deprive yourself just because it's a snail?

Well, a blowjob is the same, so stop over-thinking it. If you love cunnilingus but you don't do this for your man, how selfish are you? Blowing your man can be very erotic and bring you pleasure just by the ecstasy that you bring him.

For a lot of people, oral sex is their greatest pleasure. Some women can't orgasm if they aren't stimulated orally. While most men certainly can climax without oral sex, it's very pleasurable to many. I can't say I know any men who turn down blowjobs.

Good technique is key. The best place to start if you've never given one is by asking him. Tell him you want to try and could he please let you know what feels good. If sex partners felt comfortable in communicating with each other, everyone's sex lives would improve greatly!

A blowjob starts out with kissing his member. If you're a good kisser, BJs will come easier. A sensual kiss placed on the head of his penis will get things started. Now start to lick and gently suck his penis, starting with the head. Slowly take the head into your mouth; tease him and make him want more.

Make sure to hold his penis by the shaft and don't apply too much pressure. Gently hold and slowly stroke him, as if you were giving him a hand job. Make sure you apply your lips and tongue as a buffer; you don't want to scrape his delicate skin with your teeth. OUCH!!! The skin on his penis is sensitive, so teeth could scrape and feel rough. This will kill the mood. Your lips and tongue work as a buffer and padding.

After sucking on the head, swirl your tongue around it and lick the length of the shaft – slow long licks, and then back up to the head. The underside of the penis is very sensitive, so attention here is key.

After sucking for a bit, take the full measure of his penis into your mouth while gently massaging his balls and still stroking him. If he is very large, take in as much as you can. If you can deep throat him, go for it; he'll be very appreciative and impressed. Moving your mouth up and down on his shaft will get him going. The amount of pressure will change once he starts to build. When you know he is ready to pop, a firmer grip could slow his orgasm, making his climax very intense.

If swallowing is something you can't handle, finish him off with a hand job. If you can swallow, go for it, it isn't as bad as you might think. Just don't focus on it. If your man has really bad tasting sperm, let him know. It could be something he's eating.

As you become an expert at this, applying greater pressure to his shaft as he starts to climax will be something that will drive him crazy. Discuss this with your man and see how he likes this technique.

Enjoying oral sex is one of many pleasures that you can give each other, so enjoy!

10

AIN'T GOT NO "GAME"

This chapter is for those of you just getting into the game of sex, or who have tried but you feel like you're doing everything wrong.

First of all, what is "game"?

It's basic slang used among young people to describe interactions with women, or any interaction. If a guy is really getting it on successfully with the ladies, you'll hear the term "he's got game." Whatever he's doing is getting the job done. He's a smooth operator in the dating arena.

Some men are gifted and know how to handle themselves with just instinct. Some men are nervous and say and act like complete morons around women. Why is this?

So much about "having game" is confidence. The confidence to be you starts with trusting yourself.

Trust that you're comfortable with you and what comes out of your mouth. Try saying your lines out loud at home, and if they sound so corny or boring that even you're turned off, find some new lines.

Don't try to play another guy's game. What may come off smooth for one guy may be a disaster for you!

Don't repeat yourself. If you give a lady a compliment, say it once and move on. While women love to be complimented, continuing to say it over and over is a sign you have nothing else to say, or that it's just one of your lines. So be original. I can't express this enough!

Too many compliments also comes off a bit creepy. I had a guy at one of the gyms where I trained who was always giving me compliments, and after a while I asked management to ask him to leave me alone. He wasn't giving me sincere compliments, he was coming on to me. I wasn't interested, so it felt strange and uncomfortable.

Men are not the only creatures on earth with an ego, but when they're in the company of women some men start to brag. If you're successful, it will show in so many ways that you don't have to spend the whole evening telling her your success story. Anyone who spends time building himself or herself up comes off insecure and needy. This is a turn-off with either of the sexes.

Women love a man who's confident and

sincere. If you're successful and talented, this will shine through if you handle yourself right. Your manners, grammar, hygiene, personality, and clothing selection are all things women observe. If you have all this going for you and nothing seems to be happening, it can only be your approach.

Not everyone has a great body, looks, money, or the gift of gab – but these are the best traits to have if you want to have your game on. So let's discuss those of you with none of the above.

First impressions are important for many reasons. It can take you to second base or slam-dunk you.

Go back to basic hygiene and make sure that's covered.

If you have no style for clothes, many department stores have salespeople who will advise you on something stylish and properly fitted. Some looks are not for everyone, so try to get a second opinion.

Check out your hair – if it needs an update, go to a hair stylist and get yourself a new do. If you wear glasses and you haven't had a new pair since you were in grade school, look into new glasses or contacts. The goal here is to try and make you look current and up to date with your age group.

Having the best manners you're knowledgeable about is a plus. If manners are something that eludes you, go to the bookstore and read up. Asking a friend or relative whom you know has good manners is also an option. Good manners are a big win with the ladies; it shows good breeding, sincerity, kindness, and education.

Conversation should be spontaneous and not rehearsed, and it should be different with each person since the personalities will be different. If you find that you use the same conversation with everyone then you are in need of some "game." Relax and listen to her for a while, see what subjects she's interested in, and play off that.

On the other hand, if no conversation is happening, then maybe she's a bore, and no chemistry is going to help that.

Learn to read what people are about and it will save you so much time in the dating game. You know what you're about; you have a good idea of what you like and expect, and if you see none of this in a woman then pack up and head out. Only desperate people hang onto a relationship that just plain sucks; they stay because they believe they have no other options. If you go through life thinking that you have no other options, then you never will. Be confident and always see yourself as an asset; men who show confidence usually get what they want in life.

Try not to act goofy. If what you're about to say is immature or silly, it's best to keep quiet. Telling stupid jokes or cursing a lot might seem cool, but can be a turn-off. Don't repeat yourself or talk too much. This is hard to do when you're nervous.

Try not to ask what her astrology sign is. One-liners are so outdated. I don't know that they were ever very good, but some guys pulled them off in the seventies and eighties. Now in the next century, the ladies who fall for one-liners are most likely not going to be anyone you'll want to spend time with.

The gift of gab isn't easy to teach. You either have it or you don't. I've known some very sexy men who didn't have to do a lot of talking. They had a strong presence and confidence without being arrogant or talkative. Try to find your own style and make it work for you. We all have a style – it may need an update or a jump-start, but we all have something to offer.

Asking your lady about herself is a great place to start. It can get a conversation started and it shows that everything isn't about you. Share experiences, like travel, books you love, a TV series, or any funny topic you've shared before that worked to get a conversation started. Relax, and if conversation has to be forced, I say move on.

11

FANTASIES

Fantasies are good clean fun during sex, and the great thing about them is that even if your partner isn't into fantasies, you can have them all alone in your mind. So much of sex starts in the mind, and at times it can be what makes the experience fulfilling.

There are times when getting into the right frame of mind can be tough. This is a good time to draw from your creativity and pull up some erotic fantasy that works for you. No matter how kinky you may allow yourself to think, no one ever needs to know what drives you. These are personal and private thoughts that get you going, and that's the great thing about the mind. If you don't happen to come across a mind reader, you'll be fine.

Now for the verbal and exotic fantasies that you can share. This is a lot like mood setting, but a bit more personalized. Make sure you and your partner share the same attitudes on this subject, or you could upset the mood. You may have to experiment with a few things until you find the right subject matter for you and your partner – but just remember, fantasies can be fun and put a spark back into an old relationship that's become lazy.

Dressing up in sexy clothes is always a turn-on. Becoming a character is fun and a challenge. Costume parties are fun because for an evening you can become someone different.

Imagine this in the bedroom: ask your lady to put on a different colored wig and length. You'll be surprised how she'll transform into someone totally different. Just make sure your lady is confidant in who she is first, and a good idea is to discuss these options beforehand. I wouldn't suggest doing this with all ladies, as some could be offended and think you prefer a blond to a brunette.

Try going into an erotic shop together and pick out some fun toys or costumes. Find printed literature that you can read to each other and play off of someone else's fantasies. Watching erotic videos is also a turn-on.

Just for fun, I wrote my husband some very erotic pornography. I barely finished reading it to him before he was tearing off my nightie. He never reads porn or subscribes to girlie magazines, but the fact that I wrote it made it personal and he loved it. I'm sure in his mind he relived my words.

Bathing and showering together can be erotic. This is a good place to try oils and fragrant soaps. Bathing your partner can be very sensuous. Wash your lady's hair, massaging her scalp and neck. Bending down for a gentle kiss would be nice. After the shampoo, massage a good conditioner into her scalp and let it set while you bathe the rest of her.

Offer to shave her legs, and she may even let you continue with the shaving and put a whole new spin on things. If you were successful and she's clean-shaven, try teasing her exposed hot spots with your tongue while warm water runs down both of your bodies. I promise you she will allow you to shave her again. When the vaginal area is clean of hair, it becomes more exposed, making it easier to please. You may want to talk your lady into trying this just once for fun. I have many friends who stay clean-shaven always; their men prefer it.

If your fantasies are into the kinky *and* you and your partner agree, then go for it. Your love life is your own private business and never needs to be shared with others.

If you aren't a very sensual person, maybe having some private fun in your mind could start you down the right path. Not everyone is confident with his or her sexuality for fear of being laughed at. Trust me when I tell you we're all a little intimidated to expose this very vulnerable side of ourselves.

Learn to relax and not take everything so personally. Try to become comfortable with experimenting. If you're only comfortable doing this alone or in your private mind, then do just that. Find someone you're compatible with.

If you have the courage, go out with some really sexy person and learn from them. Sexy people sometimes don't realize they're sexy. They just go with what comes naturally. They aren't doing a whole lot of thinking, they just move with what feels good.

Try letting go. The mind is so powerful and has so much to do with sex that if you allow yourself to have erotic thoughts, you'd probably amaze yourself with what you could do.

A great example of this is if you ever had a wet dream – no one touched you, it all happened in your mind. We love having those dreams, and it's a shame we can't command them at will. Whenever you've had a wet dream, your mind took you to some great erotic thought or place and you climaxed. No one touched or stroked you, but you still had an orgasm. Sometimes you come out of the dream and don't remember what you were dreaming, but the sexy feeling is still with you. You may even drift back off and continue to have erotic thoughts.

Use your mind to conquer your sexual fears. Play out in your mind the lover you would love to be, and then try to do just that.

I've written some fantasies at the end of this book to jump-start this for you.

12

JUST GO FOR IT!

Sex is such a relaxed, sensuous moment! I think some people tend to put too much stress on it. Relax and go with what feels good.

Having an orgasm can be therapeutic. You know how some people go around with a sour face most of the time, and someone will make the comment he or she needs to get laid? What they're saying is that person is uptight and needs to chill.

You'll come across some ladies that you simply can't turn into the sex goddess you want. I call these gals the librarians. I have several male friends married to these 16th-century throwbacks, and they're miserable or cheating on them. For some reason some women feel sex requires something they simply cannot do. If you're not already married to one of these ladies, look for all the signs during dating, and if a good healthy sex life is important to you, you may want to look elsewhere. This might seem shallow, but trust me, more relationships end up in fights or breakups because someone in the relationship is tired of giving up the things they want.

Compromise can go only so far, so decide what's really important to you and try to seek those things out early in the relationship. If you just settle because there wasn't anything else going on, or you just gave up, you'll regret that decision one day for sure.

I'm open-minded enough to think that some people can change, but you should be able to spot the really prudish ones. Run, don't walk. I don't know one single situation where a miraculous adjustment was made. I've tried counseling several of my female friends that fall into the librarian category, and they just don't get it. When their only response to oral sex is yuck, what can you say?

Remember the mind and how powerful it is in sex. These ladies have already made up their minds that parts of the sexual experience are dirty, immoral, and downright disgusting. Chances are you'll never get them to change. Don't take this personally. Unless you're married, you can move on. If you're deeply in love, suggest counseling, but make sure the counselor is good with sexual situations.

My wish is that all your sexual experiences be all that you expect and more! Laugh, relax, have fun and enjoy this great gift that you have to give –yourself.

The Fantasies

THE BLACK ABYSS

The storm has been over for hours. I begin to awaken and realize I've been washed up onto some beach and can't seem to move.

I'm on a beach, and this seems like an island in the middle of nowhere. Am I paralyzed or so exhausted I can't function? I'm having difficulty remembering the events of the night before – or anything else. Where am I? Were there any other people with me? I can't remember any faces or names. There are no signs of a boat or remains of wreckage if that's how I arrived here.

My body is heavy but extremely relaxed, which puzzles me. I feel no urgency to move; lying here in the sand seems comforting. The sound of waves rolling to shore is lulling me into a hypnotic trance, and I can't fight the urge to just give in.

Smells I've never experienced are mixing into this euphoric state, but there are no signs of life, not even the sound of birds. A nice warm breeze comforts me like a warm blanket and adds to this moment of tranquility. In and out of consciousness, I'm floating in a state of peacefulness. Time does not exist, and I'm unaware of the moments passing.

I finally regain some clear thought and begin to use my eyes to search my surroundings. All I can make out is very thick foliage, lush and green with splashes of color from island flowers. Such a peaceful and beautiful place certainly deserves a name. But for right now I can't move and don't care.

Through a fog that appears with no warning, I can feel life moving in the foliage. I should be frightened, but I'm not. As vulnerable as I am at this moment, fear does not come to me. The movement in the lush green vegetation continues. I can't make out a form, but feel a very powerful presence approaching me. The fog lies over my body and all around me as if it was poured in from the sea. Slowly from the fog emerges a form: it's long and lithe and black as coal. The gentle breeze moves the fog around the body of my visitor, allowing me a glimpse. The fog seems to be pouring from the flesh of this beast and flowing down around its long sturdy legs. Its body moves in a dance with the fog, and the fog is pouring it closer to my place on the sand. I can see the glow of eyes through the mist. They glow like the sun and seem to melt the fog as the creature moves closer.

It's a cat of some kind. I can't be sure. It stands

over me exuding power, but I'm not frightened. The cat begins to smell me, nostrils flaring with the full scent of my body. My scent appears to be making it more aggressive, and it begins to lick me. The licks are erotic. The tongue is raspy, but the cat applies the right amount of pressure and the feeling of roughness with moisture sends chills over my whole body.

I have no feeling I'm to be a meal; instead, a mere toy for my new companion. With very little effort the cat's powerful jaws and teeth tears what remains of my clothes from my body until I'm exposed and completely naked.

The cat begins to lick and clean me, starting with my bare feet and slowly moving up to my loins. As it smells and licks my genitals, the cat begins to act more aggressively. My human scent is arousing this cat and it arches its powerful back throwing its head up with an explosive roar to mark me as its prey. Hot breath and licking are consuming my body. The arousal of the cat's work is evident and the cat proceeds to mount my naked form with all its black sleekness.

I am helpless and only beg that the cat continue.

Covering my body with its great black mass, a transformation begins: the cat is slowly becoming human. The cat becomes a sleek black woman with the eyes of a cat. They are yellow and mesmerizing, and I can't look away.

I feel the power of her body against me. The

heat from her body burns into my skin. If only I could touch this magnificent creature, but I cannot! My body must do all my touching for me.

She's provocatively moving her body over mine to allow me the full sensation of her powerful form. She begins to take all of my manhood into her black cave of ecstasy. I have never experienced such heat. My skin seems to be melting into this beautiful catwoman. Without any movement from my body, her black abyss sucks and pulls me into the most inviting sensation I have ever felt. I am so engorged that I begin to moan with passion. The movements are sensual and the she-cat runs her claws along my body, reminding me of the power that's taking over my being. This half-human cat creature has consumed me and is sucking me in deeper and deeper. The feeling is so overwhelming that I begin to climax, and the she-cat is following my lead. The sound of human passion and animal roars blast through the peacefulness of this oasis.

As we travel to a space of rapture her yellow eyes flare. Her glare is searing into my flesh with each convulsion of our passion.

At last we glide into a satisfied peace, and she slowly begins to move off my body. As she steps away from me she throws back her beautiful black head and roars. This powerful sound of dominance begins her transformation, and she becomes a black cat again. She slowly melts from my presence, and as mystically as she appeared from the foliage she is gone, swallowed into the fog.

A gentle breeze comes through the window and blows the folds of the mosquito net. The sun is beginning to rise and its warm rays fall on the floor of my room. Slowly the sun creeps onto the bed. I feel the warmth hit my feet and ever so slowly move up my legs. The warmth is arousing and I can feel myself becoming hard. The heat of the sun is taunting me and I can't resist its gift. As the warmth moves to my groin, the heat of the sun sends my seed spilling onto the sheet. The feeling of passion slowly leaves my body and I begin to awaken. I am confused but content. As I throw the sheets from my naked form, I am further perplexed by the long claw marks on my body.

If only sleep would come to me once more, my fantasy could begin again!

WET DREAM

THE EXECUTIVE

I followed her closely with my eyes as she entered the room. If I possessed artistic talents, I'd be able to sketch her nude body – in detail – because I'd pictured her naked so many times. In my mind I knew every line, every curve, and I'd even placed a mole underneath one of her full, round breasts. I only hoped it would look as I'd imagined, should I ever get the chance. Her legs would run up and form into a full, round, tight, and inviting behind. By the way her suits hugged her body, I knew her waist was slim and flat.

Besides her emerald green eyes, the first thing you notice are her breasts. They command everything that she wore, though her look is always clean and professional. She's the only woman I know who can make a conservative suit scream with sex appeal.

If I only had one minute with her, it would be to devour her lips. They are full and just wide enough, the kind of lips that when she speaks, you become hypnotized with every word they form. I try very hard not to be obvious with my gaze, as I've seen so many other men just staring and making her uncomfortable.

She carries herself with grace and confidence, letting the stares go unnoticed. Her position in the company comes with power. She runs this division. Most of her employees happen to be men, and I am the most junior. I'm 27 and she's 40. The age doesn't matter to me. I have never desired any woman so much in my life.

She begins the meeting and I have no idea if I can concentrate. Her mouth moves and all I focus on is the fullness of her lips. I can feel myself starting to get hard. The conference table gives me privacy.

I must gain composure and remember where I am. She's calling my name, bringing me back to reality. I look up and stare into her large green eyes. They're such a contrast to her pale skin and long dark hair. I am melting, but I have to find my brain to answer her questions. I am grateful that I've been very successful in my new position; she's singing my praises. "If she really wants to thank me," I think, "let me feel her lips on mine for just a moment." I have never felt so overwhelmed by the presence of one woman in my life.

The meeting is finally over, and I can go back to my office and away from this delicious distraction. I dive as hard as I can into my work, hoping to distract myself from the image of her in my thoughts.

At last I lean back in my chair to stretch. I have worked so diligently, I have no idea what time it is. It's dark outside. I open my office door. Everyone seems to have left, and very few lights are on in the office. I stumble down to the lunchroom and open the refrigerator, hoping for a cold soda. I pop the top and take a long swallow.

I decide to take off my tie and jacket and for the first time today I relax. Now that I am free with my thoughts again, I can think only of her.

Sitting back in the chair, I start to unbutton my shirt and kick off my shoes. My thoughts take me to the greatest desire I have. I begin to get hard, and since no one is around, I don't care. I let out a small moan of relaxation and fantasy release.

I feel someone over me and open my eyes to see her staring down at me. She points with her eyes toward my very large erection and says, "Is that for me or because of me?"

My mind shuts down. I can only act. I slowly stand up, exposing my erection even more. She seems to glow with the thought of my arousal. No words are spoken. Her body language talks to me, and I know an invitation is being offered.

I slowly move toward her and put my hand on the small of her back. Pulling her to me, I finally feel the lips I've desired for so long. Our kiss is warm and soft; we kiss with all of our bodies. She moves closer into me and feels the fullness of my erection. She's swaying and pushing her breasts into my chest. My erection is so hard I feel it may burst through my pants.

I gently pull her jacket over her shoulders and let it drop to the floor. She's wearing a silky blouse that allows me to feel her fullness even more against my body. As we kiss, I begin to pull her blouse free of her skirt and run my hands up her back. Her skin is like the silk I've imagined a thousand times.

I unfasten her bra and bring my hand around to cup her luscious mounds. She moans and lets me know I can move further. I unbutton her blouse and let it drop. I have to step back and gaze for just a moment. The desire to have one of her nipples in mouth stops my gaze and I feast on her scent and erect nipple.

She starts to unbutton the last of the buttons on my shirt. Now that our upper bodies are naked, we begin to kiss even more passionately, allowing flesh on flesh to be our tease. The feeling of her softness is driving me crazy. I push down her skirt, dying to view the rest of my fantasy. As her skirt falls to her stiletto heels I realize she is wearing no panties, and thinking that all the times that I saw her she had no panties on makes me insane.

She's more beautiful than I even imagined. The soft patch of hair between her long and luscious legs is like a black jewel. I can see the moisture of our passion glisten and run down her leg. I fall to my knees and begin to lick and tease her gently. She is moaning and grinding into my mouth. I can feel and taste her orgasm starting to build. I move my fingers into her cleft and continue to tease her bloom with my tongue. She is frantic now with passion and begins to climax. Her body is moving in a sultry spasm and her screams of passion echo through the empty offices. I slowly stand up, still holding her heat in my hand.

She can barely stand and falls into my body. Her head comes up and kisses me with a passion I have never felt. I feel her unzipping my pants and push them down. Next my underpants fall and all that I have to offer comes falling out.

Taking my penis into her hand she pulls me over lo the lunch table and pushes me down. Once she has me positioned, she begins to mount me, taking me slowly inside her heated cave. I melt into walls of velvet. She sits up and I am in awe at the beauty of this woman. As she slowly moves up and down, I can feel her heat pouring over me.

She gently falls onto my body, searing my flesh with her breasts. She grinds into me and kisses me with eagerness. I have held back as long as I can and begin to fill her cavity with a long-awaited passion. She begins to explode once again which only heightens my erotic lust. Our bodies glide slowly into a feeling I have felt in my mind a thousand times. The moment lasts longer than I have ever experienced, and I feel completely drained. She collapses onto to me and we maintain this moment for a few seconds; then she moves off of the table and me. Picking up her clothing she leaves the lunchroom as quietly as she had entered it.

Our bodies did all the communicating, and I only hope they will speak again soon.

THE HOUSEKEEPER

During my senior year of college I was struggling financially, so I decided to take up some small jobs to increase my very small income.

Since the hours were flexible, I decided to do some housekeeping. I've always been very neat and organized, so I thought cleaning for others should be an easy job. I posted some ads on campus and on social media.

After about a week, I received a call from a woman who said she needed housekeeping and some help organizing her husband's office. I went for the interview and was pleasantly surprised at how wonderful the house was. These people obviously had money, so paying me wouldn't be an issue.

Once I met the lady of the house, it got even better. She was very attractive with a pleasant smile and a quiet personality. We discussed my responsibilities and my salary. She explained that her husband worked from their home, while she worked outside the home. There were no children or pets. Sweet. I was to start the following Monday, which met with my schedule. She explained how to enter the home, since she would be away and her husband would be busy working and not available to welcome me in.

I arrived right on time and got busy doing the things she had requested. This was a very large house, so I had made an outline to address all the key areas.

I'd been there about three hours when I decided to check the husband's office. She'd said it usually required organization and cleaning. The door was ajar and I heard no voices, so I gently pushed the door open to see if Mister was at work.

As the door opened, I saw him seated at his desk looking at his computer. Whatever he was looking at had his undivided attention. I suddenly realized he was breathing very heavily – whatever was on the screen had to be juicy. Then it hit me that he was looking at porn!

When he realized he wasn't alone, without thinking, he jumped up. Well, I was shocked to see the biggest penis I have ever seen. It was throbbing and dripping from his excitement. He noticed my gaze and quickly sat down. I'm sure I was red from head to toe, but for some reason I was glued to the floor where I stood.

Thankfully, he spoke first and apologized for his situation. My mouth wouldn't work properly at first, but finally I introduced myself. He said he knew of me from his wife. He had been so engrossed in work and other activities and he hadn't paid attention to my presence in the house.

When we both had time to gather ourselves, he began to explain his situation. He said that since he was so greatly endowed, it was rare that he and his wife had sex. She just couldn't handle him, and wasn't well versed in sexual activities. So he got relief from porn.

I was shocked and confused that he would share this with a total stranger. I had no idea how to respond, so I asked if he needed my help in his office. He seemed grateful for the change of subject and started to give me some duties. As I began to clean his office he left to get lunch in the kitchen.

As I cleaned I could not get the image of his amazing cock out of my head. I realized I was turned on and getting very wet. What was wrong with me? I could not be fantasizing about this man! He was tall, drop dead handsome, and, let us not forget, *married*. I needed to focus.

As I came around to clean by his desk, I noticed he'd left the computer screen on, and the porn site was right there. The site he was on showed very large breasts and the pinkest pussies I have ever seen. Women were licking each other and men stroking their cocks while watching. Well, this set me off more than I already was. For some reason I started to rub my crotch just to try and calm myself down. My jeans were soaked.

I was so in my moment I didn't realize I had company. Mister spoke to me in the sultriest voice ever, saying, "Would you like some help with that?"

I couldn't speak, I just acted. I unzipped and dropped my jeans to the floor. As I kicked out of them, he came around the desk and began to pull my thong panties slowly down my thighs. I hadn't noticed that my juices were dripping down my legs. He bent down and started to lick and lick and lick until he got to my hot spot. When his tongue hit my throbbing pussy I exploded into an ecstasy of spasms and moans like nothing I have ever experienced. My climax lasted and lasted and until I collapsed into his arms. When I could finally breathe, I whispered, thank you. He told me he had never felt such an explosion from any woman.

He gently lifted me to his lips and kissed me with so much passion that I began to convulse again. He said, "Stop, please, let me feel this intensity on my cock! It's been so long, I can't imagine it." I couldn't say no, because I wanted to feel the measure of this man and more. He pushed everything off his desk and laid me down. He asked that I please release him from his slacks. Of course there was a massive bulge waiting for me. I slowly unzipped his pants and out came the most amazing specimen of a man I have ever seen. I put as much of my hand around his shaft as I could, and he moaned like a wild beast.

"Please, let me feel you," he begged, promising to be gentle so as not to hurt me. I said, "No, hurt me, please!"

As he started to probe my throbbing entrance, I couldn't take another second of suspense. I grabbed his hips and pulled him deep into my well of passion. He was shocked at how easily I accepted his member. He slowly moved in and out of me like a master, gliding every inch he had deeper and deeper. We were both at the very brink of madness with passion, and before I could scream he exploded into me like a thunderbolt. The release of his orgasm sent me into an intensity of lust, passion, erotic thoughts, and enjoying the biggest cock ever.

He collapsed on me, breathing in my sexual aroma, and I could feel him hardening again. He picked me up and laid me on the floor of his office and began our dance of lust again.

He was overwhelmed by my ability to take his cock. It had been a long time since he had enjoyed such pleasures.

I can't wait to clean his office again!

WELCOME HOME

I was just finishing grad school before entering medical school. Studies had consumed most of my life. I've always been an intense student, allowing very little to occupy my mind or time besides my studies.

I'm 21, tall, well built, and most people think I'm handsome. I'm also shy, and I've never felt very comfortable around women. I had dated during school, but not often, and was sadly still a virgin. I masturbate often and look at porn, but I've never had the courage to move to the real thing.

I think partly this is because I'm from a very proper and conservative family. I don't think I ever saw my parents show any affection, and never heard moans of passion coming from their room. How I was produced is still a mystery!

I was heading home for the summer to my parents' summer home in the Hamptons. When I arrived no one seemed to be home, which was fine with me. A few moments alone and a swim in the ocean and pool would be just what I needed. I threw my gear in my room, pulled on my swim trunks, and headed for the beach.

I dove into the first wave and my body felt alive and refreshed. After swimming for a while, I headed back to the house and decided to jump in the pool to rinse the salt and sand from my body.

Since no one was around, I dropped my trunks and plunged in. I swam the full length of the pool underwater, and when I popped up at the other end, there stood our neighbor and my mother's good friend, Mrs. Sanders.

I've always liked her and never fully understood her relationship with my mom. My mom is a prude, and Mrs. Sanders seems like a wildfire to me. Her husband is always gone on business, and she seems lonely. For a lady of her age, and I have no idea what that was, she's extremely attractive. She's full-figured and carries it well – and it's all her, no plastic anywhere.

As I looked at her freshly painted toes, she laughed and said, "Welcome home! It looks like school has agreed with you!"

I looked up and saw her pool robe was very sheer and left very little to the imagination. I felt myself getting hard, but – no way! This was my mom's friend, this was wrong!

But my cock didn't seem to care about the

relationship and continued to grow. I certainly couldn't get out of the pool now!

Mrs. Sanders must have sensed my desire. She dropped her robe and dove into the pool, swimming over to me. The water was moving over and around her ample breasts, and I couldn't wait to hold them.

She grabbed my hand and pulled me to the shallower end of the pool. When we reached the area about four feet deep she stood up, and I gasped at the beauty of her body. She was firm, full of curves and her breasts screamed hold me, kiss me, lick me.

But I'd never been with a naked woman, and I wasn't sure what to do. She must have known, because she grabbed my arms and pulled me to stand up. Her eyes shot to my erection; she smiled and said, "Very impressive! Now let's take him for a ride!"

She moved toward me and took me into her arms and kissed me gently at first. As her body started to feel my cock against her, she became more aggressive. Her kisses were soft and passionate, and I was getting even harder.

She began to glide me to the side of the pool and pushed me against the edge. Wrapping her legs around my torso, she guided my ever-so-hard cock into her slippery well. The sensation of her heat and the water around us was incredible. She began pumping her hips up and down while I held onto the side of the pool to support our bodies.

Slick water, slick pussy, rock hard cock – a recipe

for euphoria! The harder she pumped, the more I was about to lose control, and then she tightened her pussy around my shaft with such intensity that I could not hold off my climax any longer. I exploded into her and she exploded all over my throbbing cock. Together, we drifted into the space where only lovers travel.

As we started to ease and she slipped off me, I couldn't speak or move. She pulled me from the edge and started to drift us to the deeper end. When we were about chest deep, she reached down and began to stroke me back into form. It didn't take long! She wrapped her legs around my waist and allowed her pussy to once again devour me completely. We were weightless in the water, so our movements were effortless. We drifted deeper and deeper in the pool and into her abyss.

We once again culminated at a level I had only imagined. Since I was a virgin, I had only my masturbation to compare, and this, this was blissful.

I slowly swam us to the edge with her still wrapped around me and lifted her to the poolside. Water dripped off her beautiful breasts, legs, and the soft cloud between her legs. I started to get hard again, and decided I wanted to take this amazing woman on dry land. I carried her wet body to my bedroom and explored my welcome home gift.

A BLOW AND A BUZZ

Leaving the office and riding home, I can feel the stress of the day easing from my body. It had been an extremely demanding day, and I can't wait to get home and enjoy a glass of wine and silence.

Stepping off the elevator into my penthouse, I feel a wonderful breeze coming off the ocean. The curtain sheers are flowing in a hypnotic dance with the air. Setting down my briefcase, I see a note from my wife next to a bottle of my favorite wine and a glass. I had called her from the car saying I was on my way and the totally crappy day I'd had.

The note reads, "Take off all your clothes and join me in the bathroom!" This must be her way of helping me feel better!

Naked and heading to the bathroom with wine in hand, I realize that I already feel great, thanks to her invitation. Opening the door to the master bath, I see my lovely wife in a sexy sheer top and very skimpy panties. Our oversized tub is filled with water and bubbles. Some sort of scent is wafting from the steamy water, calming my mood further. Candles are lit everywhere.

She invites me to step into the tub, where she proceeds to wash me all over with soft, soothing strokes. She massages my head with shampoo and conditioner until my scalp tingles.

After draining the tub she rinses my body clean, and gently helps me out so she can dry me off.

I drain the last of my wine and can't wait for whatever is next. She leads me to the bedroom, where she's set up a massage table with fluffy blankets. She asks me to get on the table and lie on my stomach. My penis is soft, and she pulls it back so that it's in between my legs, exposing the underside of my scrotum. I have no clue what she's planning, and I'm intrigued!

Soft romantic music is playing, and she's lighted many candles. A breeze flows gently over my nude body, and I can hear the sounds of the waves crashing to shore. Amazing sounds, smells, and peace engulf my body.

My wife starts to drop warm oil onto my back; she gently starts to rub it into my skin and then begins a more aggressive massage, removing all the tension I'd brought home from the office. I'm slowly drifting into a calm I haven't felt in quite some time.

She massages the oil all down my legs to my feet and back up. She massages it into my hair, rubbing my scalp with just the right amount of pressure to remove tension and stress. It's amazing. I can't imagine anything better.

I begin hearing buzzing sounds, but since I'm face down, I can't see what's happening. Then I feel that she's taking the head of a massage wand and touching my butt with it. Slowly she brings the head of the vibrator to my rectum. She doesn't penetrate my rectum, but vibrates all around my anal area. Then she moves the vibrating head down the shaft of my penis, which very quickly becomes hard.

She's pressing the vibration along my cock and then back around my anal area. The sensation is beyond amazing. What she's planning next I don't care, just please don't stop! My erection is full force now and starting to throb along with the vibration. It feels like my cock is vibrating harder than the wand.

When I think it can't get any more sensual, she gently rolls me onto my back, placing a cloth over my eyes to keep me intrigued. She takes my erection into her hand and starts to stroke me, and at that very moment applies the wand head to the base of my cock and rectum. As if this sensation wasn't enough, I feel her mouth swallow my cock. The feeling of lips, tongue, suction, and vibration is like nothing any man has ever experienced. I am beyond amazed at the talent this woman is using on me!

ELISABET

She goes slowly up and down on my shaft, stopping to tease the throbbing head. Swirls of tongue deliciously trace the length of me. She begins to apply more pressure with the wand as she starts to suck more intensely. The sensation is overwhelming, and I explode into the most aggressive and violent orgasm I've ever experienced. The pressure of the wand and the suction on my cock send volts of energy down and out of my feet. The sensation lasts what seems like forever. The culmination of all that has brought me here is beyond description.

When I finally gather myself, I cannot speak. I remove the blindfold from my eyes and pull my wife into my arms and hold her with a desire and love like I have never felt before. It's as if she knew what it felt like to be a man, and gave me my fantasy!

THE LAUNDRY ROOM

I live on the fifth floor of an old walk-up apartment building. The laundry rooms are down in the basement. I'm a bachelor, and I don't have much laundry. Still, I really dislike laundry day.

To make it more bearable, I go down very late at night, hoping no one is there so I can have all the washers and dryers to myself. I usually take a book and read, so I don't have to keep coming back up the stairs.

With my basket of clothes and detergent, I start down. In all my years of doing this ritual, no one else has ever been there. I guess I'm the only weirdo doing laundry at midnight. I like the peace at this time, and since I work from home my schedule is flexible.

As I walk to the door of the laundry room, I hear a washer going – and I also hear moans! I tiptoe to investigate what's going on. Peeking around the door, to my great surprise and delight I see a very hot woman rubbing her crotch against the vibrating washer. The washer is obviously off balance and moving very aggressively. I don't know if she did this intentionally, but she sure seems to be enjoying it. Her red panties are down around her ankles and she's massaging one plump breast. I'm hypnotized by this scene. Laundry day just got a lot more interesting!

I continue watching, hoping she'll have an expressive orgasm. My wish is fulfilled! She begins to shake along with the washer, throwing her head back and groaning with ecstasy. Her legs buckle under her, so she grabs the washer, her new best friend, for support.

Once she's composed, she bends down to pull up her panties – and then she sees me standing in the doorway with an erection and a smile on my face.

Her first reaction is rage for being discovered. "How could you spy on me?" she screams. I come back to reality and realize she's really pissed at me.

I come into the room and explain that I came here to do laundry, not molest the equipment. *That* was the wrong thing to say. She starts throwing her dirty laundry at me. I catch pair of hot panties in one hand and come closer to her.

"Look, lady don't be mad at me because you can't get laid and require an off-balance washer to get off."

She lunges at me and I catch her in my arms. I

hold her tightly so she can't hit me. She starts crying, and says she's just embarrassed. Like me, she does her laundry late so that she can be alone. She explains that she got bored and horny at the same time. She bursts out laughing, and I follow suit. We're laughing so hard that we forget the awkward moment.

I start my laundry and we begin talking. She just moved in, and doesn't really know anyone. We chat a bit longer and I discover she's not just hot with an amazing body; she's also easy to talk to.

At that very moment the washer starts to vibrate again. I say, "Are you going for round two?"

"Very funny," she answers. "And you seemed to like the show."

"It *was* entertaining," I answer, moving closer to her. "You know, you could just use a cock and not machinery if you like." I hope she doesn't slap me, but instead she moves right up to me and grabs my package.

"You mean this one?" My cock starts to grow in her hand.

"Yes, that very one."

"Let's see if he can outperform the washer!" she says, unzipping my pants and to release my very angry friend from his confined space. "Well, this is certainly more interesting than the washer!"

She drops her red-hot panties and jumps onto the moving washer, saying, "I think I'll have both of you!"

     I step out of my shorts to oblige my new laundry-room friend, and grab her firm rump to pull her closer to the edge of the washer. My cock is screaming for its target, but I want to tease her before giving her what we both want. I slowly trace the engorged head of my cock around her hot wet pussy. I lean in and kiss her softly at first and then with deeper thrusts of my tongue. She is aching for the full delivery, but not yet. I want to out-do the washer, so I need to let her build a bit. I put just the tip of my member in her, and she starts going mad with desire. "Fuck me now!" she screams.

     I thrust the full length of my cock into her and the machine starts to gyrate with us. She's on fire with every thrust and vibration. As the machine slows down, I grind into her hot pussy one last time, and we both explode into delirium.

     I back away from her and find dirty laundry to wipe us clean. When I touch her heat with my favorite T-shirt, she yelps out and pushes me away. Her passion is still throbbing and way too sensitive to touch.

     I guess I out-did the washer!

THE ELEVATOR

Stepping into the elevator, I can't help but notice an extremely hot black guy. He's dressed to the nines, and he fills out his tailored suit perfectly. He smells great – not overpowering, just enough to make you notice. He's tall and broad-shouldered. I've never been with a black man, but they are for sure one of my fantasies.

I'm average height with a tight body, long blond hair and deep green eyes. I'm not in a relationship, but this doesn't bother me.

I move into the elevator and push the button for the 11th floor, and notice my black fantasy is going to the same floor. Nice.

As the door closes and we begin our climb, the elevator makes a very odd sound and jolts a bit. I think nothing of it, until I notice that we're no longer moving.

I turn to my elevator companion. "What was that?"

"I'm sure it will start back up soon," he says.

We stand there quietly for about ten minutes. Nothing is happening. I start to panic. I'm claustrophobic, and while I'm fine as long as I know that we will reach a destination, standing dead still is not comfortable.

We both decide to push the emergency button, but nothing happens and we are for sure stuck.

Tall and chocolate notices I'm starting to panic a bit. "Are you OK?"

I shake my head and explain my issues with small tight places. If we don't get out soon, I may freak out. He has a bottle of water and offers me some to try to help me calm down. It helps a bit, if only because it's taken my mind off the situation.

I take off my jacket and shoes to cool myself off, because when I panic, I get hot. This gorgeous stranger is soothing and kind, but nothing is helping.

"What can I do?" he asks. I'm starting to panic even more, which is making him nervous. Since his words aren't working, he grabs me and pulls me in for a kiss. He kisses me hard at first and it's a shock; then he takes my face into his hands and kisses me passionately. It's the most amazing kiss I've ever had in my life. He smells great, dresses well, and kisses like no man ever. I've lost my ability to breathe, and then he pulls away.

"I'm sorry, I didn't know what else to do." he says. "You were so nervous, I thought if I could take your mind off of the cramped space, you'd relax."

I still can't find breath to speak, so I just nod. Finally I can function, and all I can say is, "That was the best kiss I've ever had!"

He smiles and moves closer to me, taking me into his arms and kissing me again with passion and heat. I melt into his body and kisses. The smell of him is so intoxicating, I've forgotten about the elevator. As we kiss harder and longer, I can feel his erection against my thighs – it's a very nice bulge. I'm so hot with desire for this man, and he can sense how turned on I am. He starts unbuttoning my blouse. He drops it off of my shoulders, exposing my sexy black bra. My breasts are pouring out of the top of my bra, and he bends down to kiss my cleavage. His hands go around my back to unfasten the hooks, and out fall my breasts right into his hands.

He massages my breasts while kissing me with such heat, and then drops his head down and takes my hard nipple into his mouth. This man has the most skilled mouth! From kissing to sucking, his talents are mind-blowing.

We're both aroused and wanting more. He pulls up my skirt and cups my butt with both hands. He moans and comments how he loves my ass. His bulge is huge and about to burst out of his slacks. He moves my panties down and they fall to the tops of my feet. I kick them aside, and then I push him back, saying, "I need to see and not just feel whatever your pants are holding in!"

I undo his belt and unzip his pants, pushing them down past his hips. He is wearing boxer shorts, and out comes the crème de la crème of cocks. I can only stare at his awe-inspiring member. I take him into my hand and can't believe the weight of him. I drop his boxers down to get an even better look at him.

I start stroking his cock, and he grows even larger. He pushes me back against the wall of the elevator and lifts me up and brings me down onto his throbbing cock. I am so wet I slide right onto him and let out a groan. He's filled me to the core, and I can't get enough of him.

He moves in and out of me with long slow strokes. I am dying with passion, and can't wait any longer as I start to burst onto his shaft. I scream, "I'm coming," and he says, "I'm right behind you." We both convulse with an intensity that shakes the elevator. As we start to come back to reality we hear a loud buzzer; the elevator is about to start up.

We quickly move into action to compose ourselves, not knowing how long we have. We're fully dressed when the doors open on the eighth floor to allow people to get on.

Finally we reach the eleventh floor and step off. He turns to me and says, "Are you ok?"

"OK? I've never been better, and I think you

cured my claustrophobia!" I answer, and we both burst out laughing.

He says, "I'd like to see you again."

We exchange numbers ... and fast-forward through time – we've been dating for a year. Every now and then we get on an elevator and deliberately stop it and re-live our greatest fantasy!

***

Thank you for reading my book. I hope it helped you discover your sexual potential.

Having great sex takes time, work and patience. Communication is so important in all things. Don't allow your ego to get in the way. Explore, have fun, and love like it's your last day on Earth!

ABOUT THE AUTHOR

Elisabet is creative, funny, and caring. Over the years, she's been a resource of sex-life advice and counsel (and sometimes comfort!) for her women friends. When her men friends started asking for tips on spicing up their sex life, she decided she needed to write this book. She hopes women will read it for themselves and give it to their men, leading to a revolution of better sex and more fun for everyone!

Made in the
USA
Middletown, DE